Fibromyalgia

All You Need to Know About Fibromyalgia Including Signs and Symptoms, Remedies, Treatment and Reducing Pain and Inflammation!

Copyright 2015

Table of Contents

Introduction 1

Chapter 1: What is Fibromyalgia? 2

Chapter 2: Risk Factors, Tender Points and Diagnosis 6

Chapter 3: Treatment Strategies for Fibromyalgia 10

Chapter 4: Non-Drug Therapies for Fibromyalgia 14

Chapter 5: Cognitive Behavior Therapy for Fibromyalgia Patients 24

Chapter 6: Natural Treatments for Fibromyalgia 27

Conclusion 28

Introduction

I want to thank you and congratulate you for downloading the book, "Fibromyalgia".

This book contains helpful information about Fibromyalgia, what it is, and the signs and symptoms.

You will soon learn how Fibromyalgia is diagnosed, and the usual plan of action that a doctor will take. If you think you may currently be suffering from Fibromyalgia, this book will help you to determine if your suspicions are true, and will explain the usual treatment methods to you.

This book includes great tips about the treatment options for Fibromyalgia, and how you can get relief. This includes the different medications that your doctor may prescribe, alternative therapies that have proved to be effective, and also some self-help strategies that can be implemented alongside other treatments.

Fibromyalgia can be an extremely difficult condition to live with. Continue reading to help determine the different ways in which you can finally gain relief!

Thanks again for downloading this book, I hope you find it to be helpful!

Chapter 1:
What is Fibromyalgia?

Fibromyalgia is a medical condition characterized by widespread musculoskeletal pain, with fatigue, memory, mood, and sleep issues. The term *fibromyalgia* is derived from the Latin word *fibro* (fibrous tissues) and the Greek words *myo* (muscle) and *algia* (pain).

In layman's terms, it means widespread pain in your muscles. This disorder causes many other symptoms, and laboratory tests do not usually validate the condition. In fact, results often make the patients feel like they are hypochondriac.

Doctors usually diagnose fibromyalgia by pressing on the identified tender points, but still this method does not give a clear explanation as to where the symptoms are coming from. However, researchers are convinced that fibromyalgia amplifies painful sensations that in turn affect the way our brain processes the pain signals.

Patients suffering from fibromyalgia would describe their symptoms as similar to a flu-like infection. They often complain about extreme exhaustion. They have trouble sleeping and when they do get some sleep, they often wake up to an aching body. The symptoms often start after undergoing surgery, after a physical trauma, psychological stress, or infection.

In some patients, the symptoms accumulate over time without a particular triggering condition. Some research shows that women are more likely to develop the condition than men.

Fibromyalgia Signs and Symptoms

Patients complain of a variety of symptoms, which can cause a lot of confusion with other medical conditions. It is important to learn more about the symptoms in order to know how to manage them effectively.

Here are the two most common symptoms of the fibromyalgia syndrome:

- *Widespread pain* – The pain that is associated with the condition is often described as a dull and constant pain that lasted for a minimum of three months. To categorize the pain as widespread, a patient has to feel it on both sides of the body, and above and below the waist.

- *Chronic fatigue* – This is one of the most common symptoms of fibromyalgia. However, the fatigue associated with this condition is nothing like any normal fatigue that you may have felt before. When you have the feeling of weakness and exhaustion associated with fibromyalgia, it is highly likely for you resort to social isolation, and eventually succumb to depression.

Fatigue associated with fibromyalgia often coincides with anxiety, depression, and extreme mood swings. As a result, people with fibromyalgia have trouble sleeping. Sleep and rest do not alleviate fatigue, and the pain is usually felt around the joints in the hips, back, shoulders and the neck. Since this causes people to develop sleeping disorders, their daytime activities and feelings are gravely affected.

Other symptoms:

- *Abdominal pain*
- *Chronic headaches*
- *Depression and anxiety*
- *Inability to concentrate* – This is often referred to as "fibro fog".
- Feeling of dryness in the mouth, eyes, and nose
- *Incontinence* – The lack of control. Associated with fibromyalgia is urinary incontinence, which is the loss of bladder control - meaning you can't help but pee in your pants.
- *Irritable bowel syndrome* – This refers to the common disorder that affects the large intestines or the colon. It can cause cramping, bloating, abdominal pain, diarrhea, and constipation.
- *Painful menstrual cramps* in women
- *Hypersensitivity to heat and cold*
- *Feeling of numbness in the fingers and feet*
- *Restless legs syndrome*
- *Tender points*
- *Morning stiffness*

Causes

Doctors and researchers still do not know the exact causes of fibromyalgia, but they are made to believe that different factors are "working together" to contribute to the condition. These factors are:

- ***Genetics*** – Fibromyalgia may run in families. Some studies prove the presence of genetic mutations that are more susceptible to developing the disease.

- ***Infections*** – Doctors found out that there are illnesses that may trigger the condition or even aggravate the symptoms.

- ***Emotional / physical trauma*** – Doctors and researchers have discovered a link between post-traumatic stress disorder and fibromyalgia.

Chapter 2:
Risk Factors, Tender Points and Diagnosis

Medical researchers and scientists are convinced that repeated nerve stimulation triggers changes in the brain of someone suffering from fibromyalgia. The change is characterized by an abnormal increase of certain chemicals that signal pain in the brain, referred to as neurotransmitters. They also have reason to believe that the pain receptors in the brain develop a "database of pain memories", and these receptors develop extreme sensitivity, thus sending "exaggerated pain signals".

Risk Factors

- ***Gender*** – It was mentioned in the first chapter that fibromyalgia affects more women than men.

- ***Family history*** – If a relative or family member is suffering from the condition, then chances are higher that you will develop fibromyalgia as well.

- ***Rheumatic disease*** – If you are suffering from rheumatoid arthritis or the more life threatening lupus disease, then you are at risk of contracting fibromyalgia.

Tender Points

What are the tender points? They are localized areas of tenderness found around the joints, but they are not the joints themselves. These areas hurt if you press them with your fingers.

These tender points are not deep areas, but rather superficial, just under the surface of the skin like the area over your elbow or shoulder.

They are also small, usually about the size of a penny. They are more sensitive compared to the nearby areas. As proof, even the gentlest of pressure applied to the tender points using a finger can cause immense pain that can make a person flinch. These tender points are spread all over the body, particularly around the back, neck, chest, elbows, knees, buttocks, and the hips.

The cause of the development of these tender points is yet to be known. While it may seem that these tender points could be inflamed because of the pain, medical experts and researchers have not found proof of inflammation when they run tests on the tissue.

It is also important to point out that their locations are not random. These tender points are located in areas in the body where you expect them to be. This is why many sufferers show similar symptoms.

Diagnosis

The tender points are among the considerations when you come in for examination. However, even if these tender points can indicate where you feel pain, it is still imperative that you accurately tell your doctor the exact pain you feel.

Keep in mind that there are other symptoms of fibromyalgia, so do not concentrate on the pain. You have to tell your doctor the other likely indications of the presence of the condition, such as if you are experiencing muscle pain, sleep disturbances, extreme fatigue, anxiety, depression, and more.

For your doctor to accurately determine that you are suffering from fibromyalgia, the symptoms should have been consistent for the last three months.

Diagnosis and Misdiagnosis

Fibromyalgia is one of the many medical conditions that are usually "misunderstood". Doctors still have difficulty making the right diagnosis despite the studies about the common symptoms of the illness. Fibromyalgia is still often misdiagnosed as just a common pain disorder. Because of this, many patients receive the wrong diagnosis and instead are often being diagnosed with arthritis or chronic fatigue syndrome.

In order to get the right treatment and for doctors to make the correct prognosis of the condition, it is necessary to explain your condition correctly and in detail.

Challenges in the Diagnosis

Doctors usually make the wrong diagnosis because fibromyalgia is a condition with a variety of symptoms that can also be indicative of the presence of other medical conditions. Even now, doctors still don't have a simple and specific test that will correctly diagnose fibromyalgia.

The dilemma of most patients is that they can go from one doctor to another without actually receiving a proper diagnosis. Hence, they receive medication and treatments that appear ineffective. This causes some patients to question themselves, and think that they might just be imagining their pain.

For many years, millions of sufferers were not correctly diagnosed. Doctors' conclusions ranged from depression, to lupus, to inflammatory arthritis, to chronic fatigue syndrome, and chronic myofascial pain. While these conditions share similar symptoms, they still have their own unique symptoms that can lead doctors to the right diagnosis.

Common Tests Conducted

Most laboratory procedures are not useful in diagnosing fibromyalgia. One particular blood test, referred to as FM/a, identifies markers from the immune system blood cells in patients with fibromyalgia. However, a lot of experts are not too keen on recommending this procedure because it is still not supported with scientific evidence as of today.

Physical exams are the most common method. It is also imperative that your doctor conducts additional discussion sessions in order to identify the symptoms. What is the logic behind question and answer tests? Remember that fibromyalgia is all about pain and what you feel. Your doctor will not know the exact areas of your pain, nor can they determine the extent of that pain, by merely looking at you and putting physical pressure on specific tender points.

This is the main reason why you have to be open and honest when telling your doctor where you feel the pain and how deep the pain is. This is the only way for your doctor to make an accurate diagnosis.

Chapter 3:
Treatment Strategies for Fibromyalgia

Doctors agree that the best treatment strategies to alleviate the symptoms of fibromyalgia are a combination of non-drug therapies, medications, and self-help approaches. There are three medications approved by the FDA available for patients, but there are still other over-the-counter drugs and alternative medications to use. In addition, there are therapies that target body movements as a cure for fibromyalgia. Further still, there are do-it-yourself and home remedies that patients can comfortably use at home.

Drug Medications

The main focus of the drug medications is to reduce the widespread pain that a patient experiences. However, each of these drugs works differently. There are drugs that target the nervous system in filtering out the pain, and others that work directly on the muscles to relieve the discomfort.

Additional medications that doctors prescribe are those that help correct sleeping problems and extreme daytime fatigue. There are patients who also complain about irritable bowel movement, frequent migraine headaches, and bladder discomfort, and there are drug medications that can also be provided for these.

While tender points are almost always spot on and similar with each person, the treatment plan should still be individualized because pain is not the same for two people.

Pain Medications

- **Boost brain chemicals** – Norepinephrine and serotonin work well in the brain and the spinal cord together to downplay pain-related signals. Doctors would want to increase the production of these substances so that your body will increase its threshold of pain. The FDA approves two drugs that help boost these two transmitters, namely *Savela* (milnacipran) and *Cymbalta* (duloxetine). Doxepin and amitriptyline are the other two medications that you can take before going to bed that work well as sedatives. These medications are also categorized as anti-depressants, which are also excellent for fibromyalgia-related pain.

- **Slow down the signals** – Pain signals are sent to the brain by the muscles and tissues. There are medications that are used to treat epileptic symptoms that are usually prescribed by doctors, like *Neurontin* (gabapentin) and *Lyrica* (pregabalin). These are given in order to slow down the signals sent so that they are not interpreted as pain. Likewise, these drugs reduce the impact of the signals to prevent being read by the brain as fibromyalgia pain. These two medications are also prescribed to help patients sleep better.

- **Muscle relaxants** – Fibromyalgia sufferers complain about stiffness and tightness of their muscles. Despite being well rested, their muscles just cannot completely relax. Muscle relaxants are prescribed to ease muscle tension. These include *Flexeril* (cyclobenzaprine) and *Xanaflex* (tizanidine).

- **Analgesics** – Particularly *Ultram* (tramodol), which helps alleviate pain. Mild opioid analgesics are also capable of boosting the action of brain transmitters, norepinephrine, and serotonin, thus further giving patients the relief needed.

- **Dopamine-like medications** – The brain automatically releases dopamine once pain is established to relieve any form of discomfort, so doctors might prescribe medications that enhance the production of dopamine, like *Mirapex* (pramepixole).

To Address Sleeping Problems

Another problem of fibromyalgia sufferers is that despite having a restful sleep at night, they still tend to wake up tired in the morning. Here are some medications that your doctor might prescribe:

- **Insomnia** – Drug medications like *Ambien* (zolpidem), *Trazodone*, and *Lunesta* (eszipoclone) are usually prescribed to treat insomnia.

- **Restless legs syndrome** –In order to treat limb movements while you are sleeping, doctors recommend taking low dosages of clonazepam and *Mirapex* (pramixole). It is said that about 1/3 of patients suffering from fibromyalgia show this symptom.

To Relieve Fatigue

Fatigue is considered as the second worst symptom of fibromyalgia. However, it's not the ordinary kind of fatigue that you may feel after you've done a lot of work. Doctors associate fibromyalgia-caused fatigue with low thyroid hormone levels. About 20% to 30% of fibromyalgia patients are found to have low levels of thyroid.

By ordering some blood tests, it is possible to determine your thyroid levels, and there are supplements that you can take to increase its levels. However, there are cases wherein blood tests will show normal levels of thyroid, so these are prescribed:

- *Boost serotonin production* – There are medications that are recommended by doctors to increase the production of serotonin without altering the production of norepinephrine. *Zoloft* (sertraline), *Lexapro* (escitalopram), and *Prozac* (fluoxetine).

- *Alerting meds* – These drugs work differently from prescriptions that boost serotonin production, and these include *Nuvigil* (armodafinil), *Provigil* (modafinil), *Wellbutrin* (buprorion), and *Symmetrel* (amantadine).

Chapter 4:
Non-Drug Therapies for Fibromyalgia

While drug medications are excellent in minimizing the symptoms of fibromyalgia, there are side effects that can be quite limiting. Hence, non-drug therapies can be helpful in alleviating muscle pain. There is a wide variety of movement therapies available to treat the symptoms.

Alternative treatments are quite popular because they have very few known side effects. Acupuncture, chiropractic therapy, body massage, and meditation are among the alternative options that are popular with patients. These treatments are rooted in the belief that the body can heal itself with the use of different techniques.

However, before you try these alternatives, make sure that you consult with your doctor first.

Acupuncture

Acupuncture is a Chinese medicine that uses needles. The acupuncturist inserts several dry needles into your skin at specific target points. The principle is to release high levels of endorphins by gently twisting or manipulating the needles. Endorphins are natural opioids.

(Opioids are medications for pain relief. They are known to decrease the intensity of the pain signals that are sent to the brain effectively, thus minimizing the effects of a painful stimulus.)

In addition to increasing endorphin production, acupuncture also helps remove energy blocks, thereby restoring the natural flow of energy along the specific energy channels of the body, referred to as the meridians.

There are studies that prove the ability of acupuncture to modify brain chemistry, by changing the way neurotransmitters are released. The neurotransmitters are responsible for stimulating or inhibiting nerve impulses in the brain that bring information, signals, impulses, and sensations from the outside, including pain. This process will increase your tolerance to pain, thus minimizing the symptoms of fibromyalgia.

Patients prefer this alternative treatment because the results can last for weeks, even from a single acupuncture session. There is even a study to prove this claim. There are patients claiming to have shown a decrease in the amount of pain they felt every day and how their quality of life has greatly improved since undergoing acupuncture treatments. More studies are still being conducted to further see how this alternative treatment can effectively treat fibromyalgia.

Chiropractic Care

Chiropractic care is slowly becoming one of the preferred alternative treatments for fibromyalgia. Most patients seek chiropractic treatment to relieve extreme pain in the neck, shoulders, back, and the various pressure points. It can also help relieve migraine headaches caused by fibromyalgia.

Many patients who complain of extreme pain resulting from musculoskeletal injuries attest to finding relief from chiropractic treatment.

Chiropractic care may be effective because it can reduce your body's pain levels.

Chiropractic treatment is based on the belief that pain and illnesses are brought about by misalignments of the skeletal structure. This alternative treatment views the body as a connected system relying mainly on the muscles, bones, tendons, ligaments and joints to continue functioning the way it should. When you have a healthy skeletal structure, your body will be healthy, too. However, even the slightest imbalance can cause serious medical conditions, including chronic pain, one of the most common symptoms of fibromyalgia.

This alternative treatment aims to relieve pain and other symptoms by restoring the imbalances in the skeletal system. There are several techniques, including stretching, adjustments and different manipulation that the chiropractor will perform in order to bring back the balance to your skeletal structure. This will result in the reduction or even the complete elimination of pain.

Fibromyalgia and Chiropractic Treatment

Patients have begun seeking chiropractic treatment because of its benefits. But how effective is it really?

Fibromyalgia sufferers usually have constant pain in the neck and back, and extreme leg cramps. To address these issues, they go to chiropractors to make simple adjustments to restore the misaligned skeletal system. Sufferers usually develop a condition known as upper cervical spinal stenosis. This medical condition can cause the compression of the meninges, the covering of the upper part of the spine. This results in debilitating overall pain. The chiropractor will make adjustments on the head and the neck as a means of releasing the compression, thus relieving the severe pain.

Is it an Effective Treatment?

There are studies that can prove its efficiency in relieving pain. There was a study in 1985, conducted to 81 patients to determine if they preferred drug medications or alternative treatments for fibromyalgia. While there are those who cite drugs as good pain relievers, chiropractic treatment had higher scores, proving that patients prefer this alternative technique for fibromyalgia.

In other studies, spinal manipulation is also a preferred treatment for pain. Some patients say that within just 15 sessions, they noticed a dramatic reduction in pain and fatigue. They also started sleeping better.

Two Types of Chiropractors

Should you decide to undergo chiropractic treatment, it is important to know that there are different kinds of techniques that are used in their programs. They are usually divided into two main groups:

- **"Straight"** – They are considered purists because their treatment and principles adhere strictly to the original techniques and teachings of chiropractic medicine. These types of chiropractors focus more on manipulations to relieve pain and restore the body's functionality.

- **"Mixers"** – The mixers use chiropractic techniques in combination with other holistic techniques, like massage, exercise, and diet. The majority of modern chiropractors are mixers.

Manipulations

Manipulation is considered as the most popular technique used in chiropractic care. It is the process of making adjustments to your spine and neck. The process usually consists of a short and quick thrust to one of the vertebra in the spine. This is done by making twisting and turning movements. Hand pressure can also be applied. This process will help bring back the vertebra to its correct place.

Expect to hear a popping or cracking sound when a manipulation technique is done. There are patients who fear that they might be injured when they undergo such a technique, but chiropractors can assure you that it is perfectly healthy. The process of manipulation helps release the carbon dioxide, nitrogen, and oxygen that has built up in your joints through time. When these particular gases are expelled, you will feel immediate relief. However, expect some discomfort, especially during the first session.

The benefits of manipulations are as follows:

- Increases blood flow (facilitates the release of toxins from the body and helps promote muscle healing)
- Boosts the production of endorphins (the body's natural pain killers)
- Gives a better range of motion within your joints
- Increased tolerance to pain

Are there any side effects?

Some groups put a shadow of doubt in chiropractic care because of the perceived possible dangers of "adjusting" and "manipulating" the skeletal structure. Some doctors and patients fear of blood clots and internal bleeding, which is only caused on very rare occasions. Bone fractures are also associated with manipulations, particularly on patients with degenerative conditions like osteoporosis.

Because of these possibilities, it is important that you consult with a health care professional before going into chiropractic therapy.

Choosing your Chiropractor

It is necessary to choose a qualified and experienced chiropractor because you may consider the treatment too sensitive. It may be difficult to find one that suits your needs, but the tips below will simplify the process:

- Chiropractors should have a license from the state where he/she practices their profession. There is also the National Board exams that chiropractors should pass.

- You can get recommendations from family, friends, and co-workers if they know one.

- The best thing to do is to ask references from fibromyalgia sufferers.

- Be sure to get to know the clinic first before setting up an appointment for a meeting. Have some questions about the techniques and strategies that the clinic uses for fibromyalgia patients. You have to make sure that you understand the procedure completely.

- It is important to check out their clinic or office. You have to make sure that the practitioner has a clean and welcoming office. It is important that it looks professional.

- Engage in some conversations with the chiropractor and avoid those that come off as having only one particular school of thought.

- Do not believe a chiropractor who seems to think that he/she knows how to cure other chronic conditions, like arthritis, and diabetes.

Massage Therapy

Massage therapy is good for patients with fibromyalgia. Who doesn't love a good whole body massage? Massage therapy helps you relax and loosen those tight muscles and relieve body aches and pain. It has a lot medical benefits; hence, a lot of patients include massage therapy as a part of fibromyalgia treatment.

Aside from relaxation, massage therapy can also help decrease stress and anxiety, and improves your general well-being. It also effectively releases endorphins.

What sort of body massage is good for fibromyalgia patients? When choosing the right kind of massage therapy for you, you have to make sure that the type you choose will ease not just the physical effects of fibromyalgia, but also its mental effects. The best massage treatment is a combination of pressure, kneading, stretching, heat application, and friction to help improve circulation and expel built-up toxins within your muscles.

The following are recommended for fibromyalgia patients:

- **Trigger Point Therapy** – You should know by now that the trigger points are painful areas in the muscle fibers. Those who are suffering from fibromyalgia have more trigger points than those who do not have the condition. The purpose of trigger point therapy is to deactivate the trigger points with the use of finger pressure. When these trigger points are properly identified and the needed pressure is applied, pain and discomfort associated with fibromyalgia are relieved.

- **Swedish massage** – This technique is popular because it is a combination of various techniques: beating, friction, kneading, and sliding/gliding. All of these techniques promote proper circulation. Patients suffering from fibromyalgia usually suffer from stress, and a Swedish massage can help relieve this stress and make them relax.

- **Myofascial release** – This process applies gentle sustaining pressure to your connective tissue. It can effectively relieve pain caused by fibromyalgia. It also restores regular motion by elongating muscle fibers.

- **Hot stone massage** – Heated flat stones are placed over the key points in the body. It has relaxing benefits and helps ease fibromyalgia symptoms.

- **Stretching** –Patients benefit from passive stretching because they have stiff joints as a result of constant muscle spasms caused by fibromyalgia. Stretching involves applying external force on your limbs to bring to a "new position". Gently stretching the arms and legs in the same direction helps loosen the stiff muscles and joints.

- **Sports massage** – This type of massage is used before or after any form of sporting event. However, doctors also recommend this technique to fibromyalgia patients. Some of its benefits are stress and tension relief, lowering of blood pressure, improved circulation, increased lymph flow, and improvement in flexibility and pain relief.

How to Maximize the Benefits of Massage Therapy

It is important that the therapist knows your condition because when you are suffering from fibromyalgia, it is necessary for your therapist to apply utmost care when applying pressure. This is why deep-tissue massage is not recommended for patients because its main focus are the muscles located deep beneath the surface.

Before getting a massage, make sure that you consult with your doctor first. If your doctor approves of it, then you have to look for a reputable therapist, particularly one that has handled fibromyalgia patients. You can check out your local hospital or a medical facility because clinical massage therapists working in hospitals are likely to understand what happens to the body when you are suffering from fibromyalgia. Do not go to the traditional spa and massage parlors because the therapists may not know what the condition is all about.

You can ask your doctor for recommendations, too. It is best if you can find a massage therapist from the hospital because your doctor can directly talk to him/her in case the therapist is not familiar with your condition.

Depending on the severity of the symptoms, the therapist may suggest that you go to several sessions until the symptoms completely disappear.

You also have to make sure that there is open communication between you and the therapist. Part of your healing process is that you are able to make the therapist understand how much pain you are feeling so that a safer and more appropriate treatment plan can be put in place.

Chapter 5:
Cognitive Behavior Therapy for Fibromyalgia Patients

The main point of the treatment plans for fibromyalgia is to ease widespread pain and relieve chronic fatigue so that patients can enjoy their lives again. One non-drug treatment that is considered as effective is cognitive behavior therapy.

Cognitive behavior therapy emphasizes the importance of your thoughts in connection to what you do and how you feel. This form of psychotherapy combines two types of therapies, namely the cognitive and behavioral therapies. Cognitive therapy aims to eliminate thought patterns that influence the symptoms, while behavioral therapy helps you to create changes in your behavior that can influence the symptoms.

Your Brain and Your Behavior

Your thought patterns influence the way you feel and act; so if you are currently in stressful and challenging situations, it is important to determine what thoughts you have been having that might be causing those feelings and actions. Once the destructive thoughts are identified, it will be easier to replace them with more positive thoughts that can lead to more positive reactions.

This treatment can effectively pinpoint the emotions you feel when you are stressed due to fibromyalgia. From the treatment, you will learn how to deal with these emotions in a way that will have a lesser impact on the symptoms of fibromyalgia.

What to Expect in a Therapy Session

Sessions usually take an hour to finish. For fibromyalgia patients to get the results they desire, they have to complete at least 6 to as much as 20 sessions, depending on the severity of their symptoms and the recommendation of the therapist and the attending physician. A typical session consists of discussing the symptoms and the way these symptoms have affected a patient's way of life.

The psychotherapist discusses with you about your feelings, emotions, and attitudes towards how you view and deal with your condition. You will both be looking for connections between your emotions and the various symptoms of fibromyalgia, and find ways as to how you can deal with the changing emotions and behaviors so that they will not further worsen the symptoms.

In each session, you might learn:

- To challenge all your negative thoughts and beliefs
- To set limitations on your duties and responsibilities
- To focus on what activities that you need to prioritize
- To accept lapses and mistakes

How Cognitive Behavior Therapy Affects the Symptoms

There is evidence that shows that cognitive behavior therapy can relieve pain and fatigue caused by fibromyalgia in about 25% of patients. It has also been proven to reduce sleeping problems, including erratic sleeping and waking schedules, and conditioned bedtime arousal. It can also effectively relieve stiffness and pain in the muscles.

There is a study showing that after just 8 sessions, patients cited lesser pain and fatigue. They were also able to sleep better. Some patients also reported that in just 8 weeks of treatment, their moods changed and improved.

Psychotherapists recommend physical fitness training alongside with cognitive behavior therapy.

Chapter 6:
Natural Treatments for Fibromyalgia

Aside from drug medications and various therapies, there are several things that you can use and do to treat fibromyalgia naturally. Some of these natural treatments are covered in this chapter.

Vitamin D

Vitamin D and magnesium levels are said to decrease in fibromyalgia patients. While the effects of Vitamin supplements have yet to be clinically proven, the natural source of Vitamin D, which is sunshine, has proven effects on chronic pain associated with fibromyalgia. So, go out in the sun once in a while.

Capsaicin

Capsaicin is derived from pepper plants. It is considered as a natural painkiller. It is used as an active ingredient for lotions and sprays. Applying capsaicin into a painful area can help stimulate the release of substance P, which becomes depleted when pain escalates. The effect, however, is temporary.

Melatonin

Melatonin is a hormone naturally produced by the body. It promotes sleep. There is a pill form available and used as a sleeping aid, but it has also been shown to be acceptable for treating chronic fatigue, depression, and fibromyalgia. While there is no hard evidence yet to prove this claim, melatonin effectively helps you get some restful sleep, thus targeting one symptom of your condition, sleeping issues.

Conclusion

Thank you again for downloading this book!

I hope this book was able to help you learn more about Fibromyalgia!

The next step is to put the strategies provided into use, and begin getting relief from Fibromyalgia. Remember to always consult with a medical professional before undertaking any treatment.

Finally, if you enjoyed this book, please take the time to share your thoughts and post a review on Amazon. It'd be greatly appreciated!

Thank you and good luck!

www.ingramcontent.com/pod-product-compliance
Lightning Source LLC
LaVergne TN
LVHW021746060526
838200LV00052B/3512